CARB CYCLING COOKBOOK FOR BEGINNERS

THE ULTIMATE EASY MADE 7-DAYS WEIGHT LOSS PLAN

BY

Mildred Kent

Copyright Notice

TABLE OF CONTENT

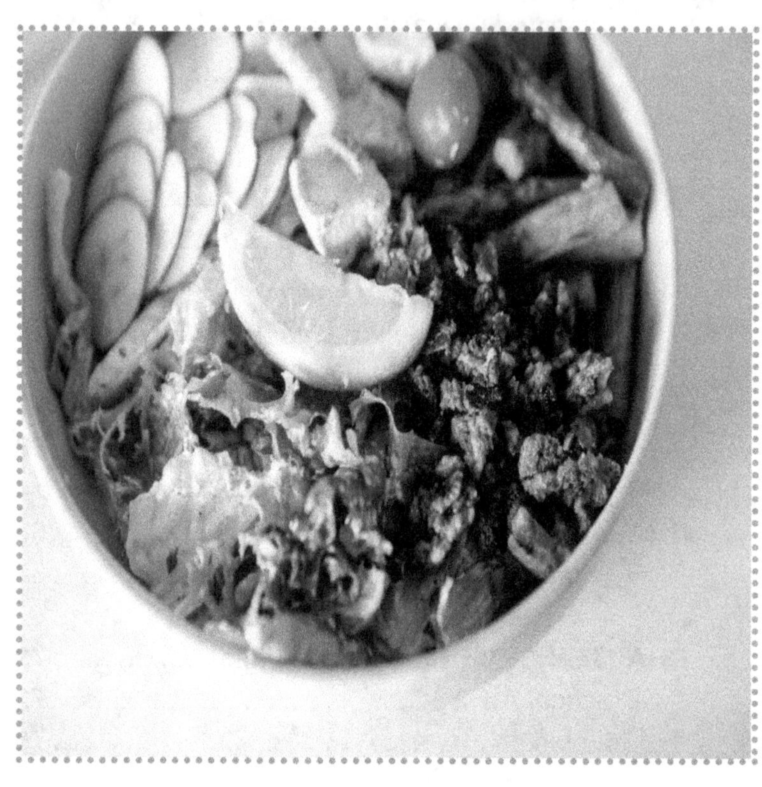

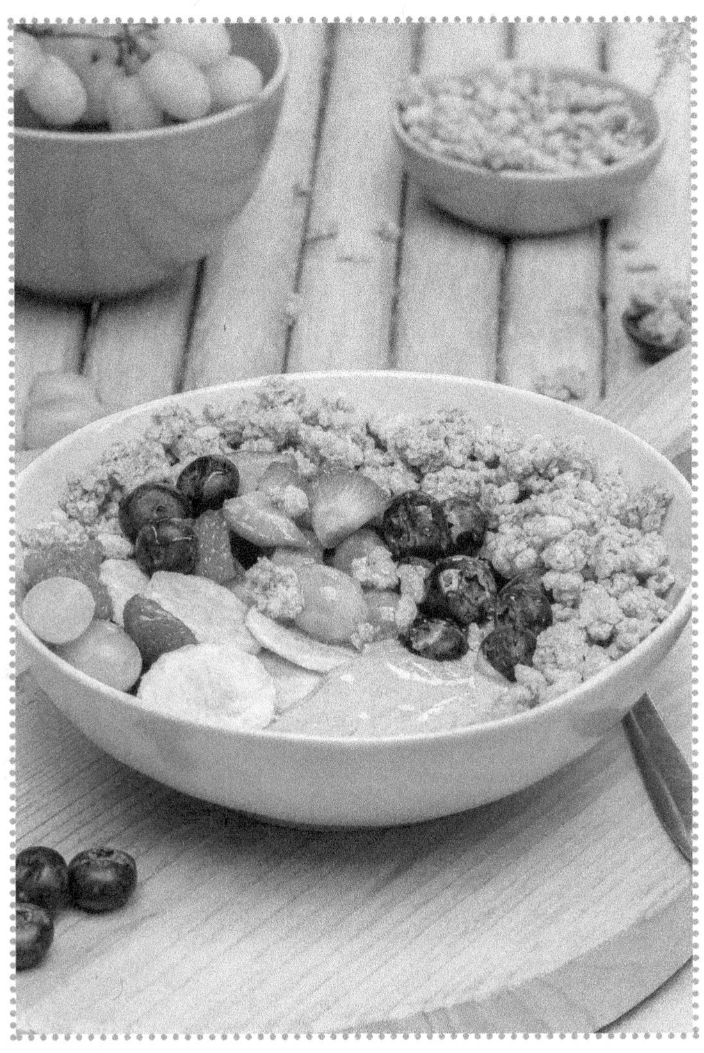

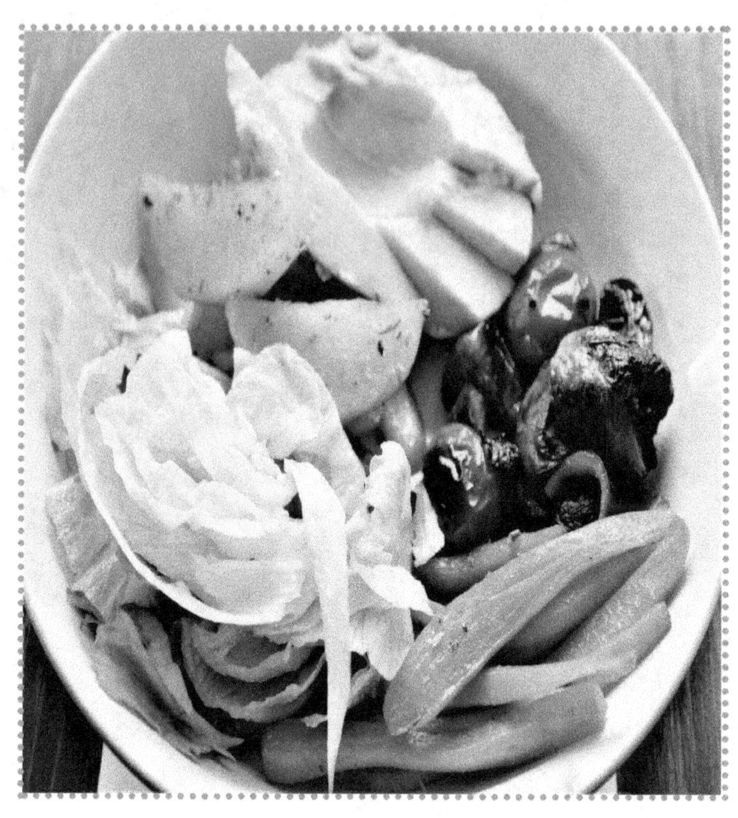

INTRODUCTION

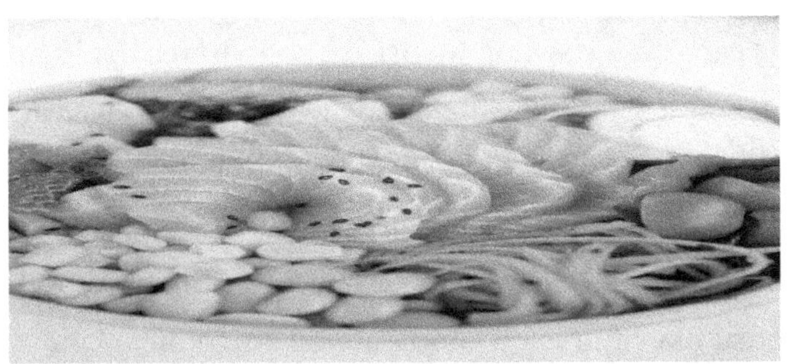

The phrase "carbs" is like heresy to anyone who is trying to lose weight. Carbohydrates are the old enemy. For Weight Watchers everywhere, carbohydrates are the wicked enemy. Carbs are high in calories, and losing weight means reducing calories.

It's a common misconception that eating a lot of carbohydrates will make you gain weight. Since whole grains and starchy vegetables are high in carbohydrates, many traditional diets also limit them. As a result, we now think that carbohydrates are unhealthy for us. They are not only harmful, but they also make losing weight difficult.

Recently, science has disproved this notion by indicating that carbohydrates might be your greatest ally while trying to shed pounds. It's known as carb cycling when we use carbohydrates to aid in weight loss. It's a way that eating carbohydrates can help you lose weight instead of gaining it!

Carb cycling is accomplished by following a weekly meal plan and a few fundamental guidelines. You have the rest of the run.

of the food you consume. You can include all of your favorite nutritious foods, including carbohydrates, in your meal plans. Even cheat days are given to you so you can indulge in your favorite, less healthful meals to sate your cravings!

What Makes the 7-Day Plan Unique?

Many of us battle with our weight and work hard to maintain a healthy, fit physique. All of us have dabbled with various eating plans and diets. We've experimented with diets that guaranteed

remarkable weight loss in X days. We've tried diets
that assured us we would never experience fatigue
or hunger. We've experimented with diets that
promised you could eat everything and still lose
weight, only to discover that "everything" really
meant spoonfuls.

We've been let down more than once. Either we
give up and binge uncontrollably, or we become too
demoralized to go on. For us, most typical diets, if
not all of them, just don't work.
What distinguishes the carb cycling regimen from
others? First of all, it makes perfect sense because it
deals with our metabolism instead of being greater
than our stomach.

Ultimately, our metabolism is responsible for
burning calories and shedding excess weight.

Second, it has long been a favorite among athletes,
particularly those who engage in intense resistance
training, despite the fact that it has lately been
heralded as a breakthrough in the fields of healthy
eating and weight loss. To increase their energy

levels and gain lean muscle mass, many of them rely on carb cycling.

Thirdly, compared to other diets, a carb recycling plan is less restrictive. As a result, it is simple to follow.

Fourthly, you have to quit the strategy after using it to reach your short-term weight loss objectives. To maintain your health and fitness for the rest of your life, you can utilize some of it to create wholesome eating habits that will last a lifetime.

For the layperson who wants to try the 7-day carb cycling strategy, this is a very basic guide. We won't delve into the finer points of how carb recycling operates, the various hormones it causes, or the intricacies of complicated measures. It will outline the steps you need to take to put together your seven-day carb cycling strategy as well as how and why carb cycling works. The outcomes will be self-explanatory.

So this book will get you started if you are thinking about trying the carb cycling strategy.

I have to add the standard disclaimer here. Before starting this plan, make sure to speak with your doctor if you have a chronic ailment or are taking any medications.

CHAPTER ONE

The Mechanism of Carb Cycling

Do you recall how old railway trains worked? The workers used to stand in front of a massive coal furnace and shovel in huge amounts of coal; the train would run at full speed if the furnace was regularly fueled; it would slow down if the coal input slowed down; and it would come to a stop if the furnace was not regularly fed with coal.

This mechanism is quite similar to the metabolism in our bodies. The primary food group that "fuels" our metabolism to burn calories and provide us with energy is carbs. Plus, carbs are quite filling. Consequently, we experience fatigue and sluggishness from diets that exclude or severely restrict carbohydrates. They also increase our propensity to binge and make us agitated and hungry.

The 7-day carb cycling regimen encourages the consumption of carbohydrates to increase metabolism. The strategy makes the body employ foods high in crab to perform at its best, burning fat and gaining muscle. Less flab and weight loss are the outcomes. It's that easy! This is what distinguishes and revolutionizes carb cycling.

There's a catch, though. This does not imply consuming excessive amounts of carbohydrates every single day. The hitch is that you have to stick to a 7-day diet where you eat fewer or no carbohydrates on some days and more on others. This enables your body to "cycle" carbohydrates in a way that promotes weight loss and muscular growth.
The idea behind this is that your body is compelled to burn fat for energy on days when you consume more fat and less carbohydrates. Losing weight is the result of this. The goal of the high-carb days is to maintain a healthy and optimally functioning metabolism, which will provide you energy.

The 7-day Plan: What Is It?

The weekly strategy switches up high-carb and low-carb days to maintain a consistent cycle of fat burning in your metabolism.
You can consume less fat and more carbohydrates on days when you're rich in carbohydrates. You can decide to eat less carbohydrates or not at all on low-carb days, but you should consume more fat and protein.

Regular exercisers and athletes frequently decide to time their high-carb days to coincide with practice or exercises when they are feeling particularly energized. On days when you are especially active, you might want to take this into account.

A typical 7-day plan looks like this:

Monday: High carb intake

Tuesday: Low carb intake

Wednesday: High carb intake.

Thursday: Low carb intake.

Friday: High carb intake.

Saturday: You have the choice to treat yourself or have a high-carb day. You are allowed to enjoy your favorite meals in moderation. This is also called "cheat day".

Sunday: Low carb day.

Versions of the 7-day plan

The strategy comes in multiple variations, some of which call for two or more days of high carbohydrate eating followed by days of reduced carbohydrate eating. Here are a few instances:

First alternative plan

Day 1: Lots of carbohydrates

Day 2: Minimal carbohydrates

Day 3: Have no carbohydrates

Day 4: Minimal carbohydrates

Day 5: Lots of carbohydrates

Day 6: Minimal carbohydrates

Day 7: No carbohydrates

Second alternative plan

Day 1: Lots of carbohydrates

Day 2: Minimal carbohydrates

Day 3: Have no carbohydrates

Day 4: Minimal carbohydrates

Day 5: Lots of carbohydrates

Day 6: Minimal carbohydrates

Day 7: No carbohydrates

There are plenty of additional variations as well, including four days with high carbs and three days with reduced carbs. But if you're just starting out, you should start with the straightforward alternate-day strategy.

When you are ready and get the hang of it, you can move to a different cycle. Alternatively, you can follow the fundamental strategy all the way through to the point of weight loss.

If carb cycling proves to be effective for you, you might want to look more closely at these additional strategies. In this situation, you should speak with an expert. They will assist you in creating a strategy that works for your gender, lifestyle, and weight objectives.

The alternate-day schedule that we'll be using here is ideal for beginners and is suitable for anyone.

What You Consume

1. The body uses carbs as its primary fuel source and needs them to speed up metabolism. They are also necessary for initiating the cycle of fat burning.

2. The basis of your carb cycling strategy is protein. Every meal must provide one-fifth to one-seventh of the daily minimum necessary intake.

3. Fats: Throughout the regimen, the amount of fat consumed will not change. On low-carb days, you may increase your fat consumption somewhat to get additional energy.

figuring out how much you consume each day

You must compute your daily intake of carbohydrates, proteins, and lipids for optimal outcomes. This multiplication technique is quite simple.

Days low in carbohydrates

1. To calculate carbs, women just need to multiply their body weight by 0.6. Male body weight should be multiplied by 0.9. The amount that emerges will be the daily consumption of carbohydrates in grams.

2. For women, the daily protein intake can be determined by multiplying their body weight by 1.2. Men can determine how much they should eat each day by multiplying their body weight by 1.5. The quantity that results represents the necessary daily consumption of protein.

3. Fats: Women should double their body weight by 0.5, and males should multiply by 0.8, to determine their daily fat consumption. The resultant figure represents the grams of fat you consume each day.

Add the totals from the three food groups to determine the overall calorie count.

Days heavy in carbohydrates

The same formula applies here, but you'll be consuming more proteins and carbohydrates. You will consume less fat overall.

1. **Carbs**: Men's body weight should be multiplied by 1.7, while women's should be multiplied by 1.4.

2. **Proteins**: Yes, the same ratio as for carbohydrates applies here: men's body weight is multiplied by 1.7 and women's by 1.4.

3. **Fats**: Bodyweight should be multiplied by 0.3 for women and 0.6 for men.
You may calculate the total number of calories you can have on high-carb days by adding the three values together.
Whether you eat three meals a day or six, the distribution of your daily consumption is entirely up to you.

Calories

The suggested range for daily calorie consumption
is 1500–2300 for women and 1500–3000 for
males. This is the general range that is advised for
you to adhere to. Don't punish yourself, though, if
you occasionally go above and above. I strongly
advise you to purchase a calorie counter app. You
may quickly find out how many calories are in the
items you eat online and create a reference list that
you can save on your computer.

Sections

On days with high carbs (200–300 grams),
amounts of carbohydrates are between 50 and 150
grams. In a subsequent chapter, we will talk about
meal varieties and portions.

This provided a very basic overview of the carb
cycling plan's operation. Let's now explore its
mechanism of action and potential advantages for
you.

CHAPTER TWO

Why the Carb Cycling Diet Is Effective

Recently, the carb cycling diet has gained popularity. Regarding the further advantages, research is currently being done. For a variety of reasons, though, a large number of people have claimed excellent success with the 7-day regimen. Here are a few justifications on why it functions:

• One of the primary causes is adaptability. With so many different items to pick from, it hardly feels like a diet. On some days, you can indulge in your favorite cuisine. Those who stick to the plan say they don't feel left out. The cheat day is also a big help!

• If you follow the fundamental guidelines, it allows you to personalize your plan.

• It's simple to incorporate into your daily routine and develop into a long-term dietary habit.

It's an easy routine to follow. The simple instructions are easy enough for even the most novice person to follow in order to lose weight.

• The fact that it has been demonstrated to burn fat and build muscle at the same time may be its best asset. Anyone who wants to lose those stubborn pounds can finally achieve their goal with this.

• It has been demonstrated that a diet heavy in carbohydrates causes the pancreas to produce more insulin. This crucial hormone increases energy and metabolism. Additionally, insulin promotes a healthier body composition.

• Eating a lot of carbohydrates causes the body to produce more leptin, a hormone that reduces appetite.

• The days with high carbs will restore and fuel glycogen, a substance that helps muscles grow.

• There's no need to track macronutrients or utilize complex measures. Simply keeping an eye on your daily caloric intake and adhering to the recommended parameters will yield effects.

 It was once thought that losing weight and gaining muscle could not be accomplished simultaneously. This is due to the fact that gaining muscle requires calorie consumption that is higher than that of shedding fat. Remarkably, glucose cycling is the secret sauce that enables the body to accomplish both. The true game-changer is this.

Because it's a healthy approach to weight loss and improving physical fitness, carb cycling is effective

CHAPTER THREE

Getting Off to a Good Start

Prior to beginning your plan, do some research to save yourself a great deal of time, trouble, and mistakes. These are the prerequisites that must be met in order to get off to a good start.

Select Your Scheme

Choose which days will be high-carb and which days will be low-carb first. We'll employ the alternating high-carb/low-carb day schedule for simplicity's sake. To utilize a different version from the ones mentioned above, simply rearrange the meal plans to align with your daily schedule.

Though it's not a requirement, ideally your high-carb days should fall on the days you're most active. Choose your "cheat day" next.

You will follow this plan for the upcoming month. It is not advised to change plans in the middle because this will break the current cycle.

Choose How Many Meals You Will Eat.

It is entirely up to you how many meals you consume in a day. Some people would rather have four or six smaller meals than the customary three. If you tend to graze more during the day, this kind of regimen might be right for you. Healthy snacks are also included in the three-meal plans. It will be more effective to eat multiple meals throughout the day if you are the kind of person that gets hungry easily.

More experienced carb cyclers might also include fasting or limit their meals to just two each day. For novices, this is not advised, though.

Decide on a weekly meal plan.

Now comes the enjoyable part! Meal planning is best done on a weekly, bimonthly, or even monthly basis if you're very organized. You won't have to deal with the stress of rushing to prepare a dinner at the last minute.

The day, the amount of meals, and whether it is a high- or low-carb day should all be listed in the meal plan.
The time you will eat each meal should come first. The times are merely a suggested structure. On days when you feel particularly hungry, you can eat a little sooner at your next meal.

Additionally, there are some hectic days when you simply cannot follow your routine. Meals can be eaten a little later, but avoid skipping them completely to avoid affecting your metabolism.

Add the serving sizes you plan to have at each meal.

Ensure You Have Enough Food on Hand

Everything you need for your meal planning should be in your fridge and cupboards. Weekly grocery shopping is a smart option if you need to buy food for everyone. Certain items can be frozen, while others can be stored so that veggies don't go bad. In a later chapter, there will be some sample meal plans to help you along the way.

Recall that you cannot switch up your high-carb and low-carb days until you have followed your selected plan for at least four weeks.

Store Up on Healthful, Long-Lived Carbs
Many nutritious carbohydrates, such as potatoes, legumes, and nuts, store well. To ensure you never run out of carbohydrates, buy them in quantity.

Suggested Portion Sizes

Some meal plans (if you are utilizing meal plans
you obtained online, for example) offer portions in
half-cups or cups in addition to the suggested
amounts for carbohydrates and calories. Everything
is OK here. Complex conversions are not required.

You'll notice that you'll consume more protein and
fat on low-carb days. Ensure that the fats and
proteins you eat are healthful.

Purchase a tiny food scale to make measuring
grams and ounces of food easy.

The recommended daily consumption of lipids,
proteins, and carbohydrates is to be followed.

HIGH CARB DAYS

**FOOD TYPE GRAMS PER
 POUND OF
 BODY WEIGHT**

Carbs	2 – 2.5 gm.
Proteins	1 gm.
Fats	-0.15 gm.-

LOW CARB DAYS

FOOD TYPE GRAMS
PER
BODY
WEIGHT

Carbs	0.5 gm.
Proteins	1.5 gm.
Fats	0.35.

After you've taken care of these fundamentals, you may move on to the next phase, which is deciding what to eat and what not to.

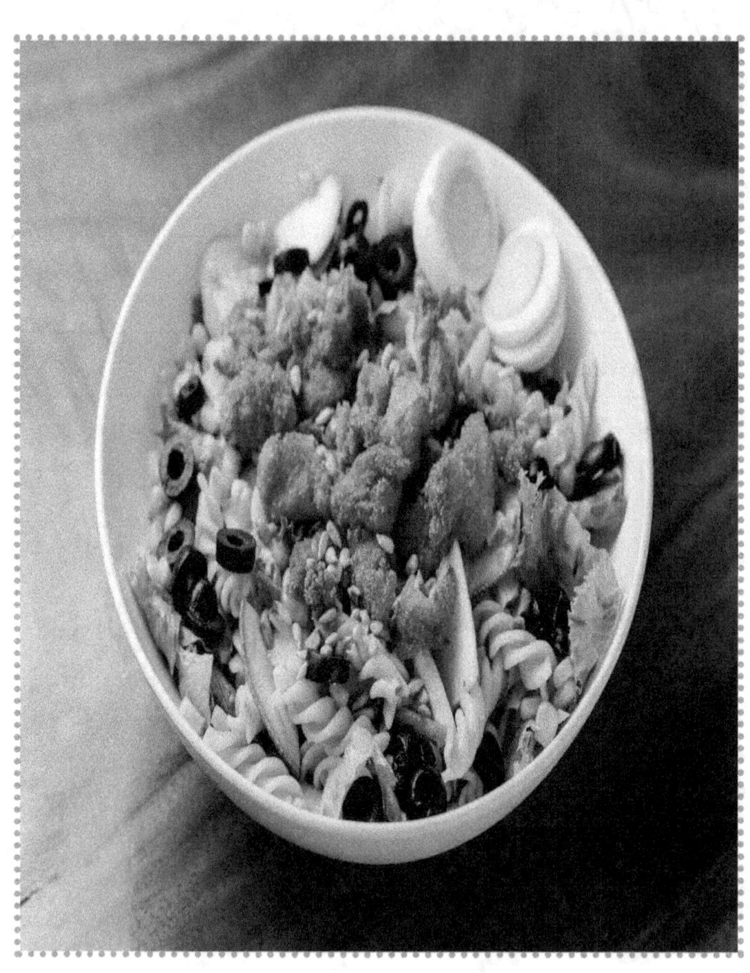

CHAPTER FOUR

FOODS TO CONSUME AND AVOID

Good vs. Bad Carbohydrates

You should, above all, consume good carbohydrates and shun bad ones like the plague. Complex or unprocessed carbohydrates are considered healthy carbohydrates. Processed carbohydrates are ones that have very little nutritional value and are packed with empty calories.

For your carbohydrate diet to be effective, you really need to adhere to this restriction. Therefore, if you have a white bread addiction, try your hardest to resist it—maybe having a slice on cheat days. Fortunately, there is something on the list of nutritious carbohydrates for everyone because it is so diverse.

HEALTHY UNPROCESSED CARBS	UNHEALTHY COMPLEX CARBS
Brown rice Natural sweeteners like honey or molasses Whole grain bread Whole grain pasta	White or whole wheat flour Table sugar
Sprouted grains like buckwheat, oats, and quinoa White potatoes Sweet potatoes Lentils All types of beans	Processed cereals Store-bought cookies and cakes Soft drinks Pizza French fries

and legumes Butternut squash Oatmeal	white pasta Muffins
Corn Peas Couscous Carbohydrate-dense fruits like bananas, peaches, plums, pineapple, and blueberries Beets Some vegetable with low amounts of carbs include tomatoes, mushrooms, cabbage, Brussel sprouts, and peppers.	Tortillas and wraps Processed chips and similar snacks Ice cream Jams and jellies Processed fruit juices Pretzels and bagels Chocolate and candy Pancakes Beer

Good vs Bad Fats and Proteins

The main components of your low-carb days are vegetables, proteins, and fats. However, the whole point is lost if you're eating unhealthy fats and proteins throughout your low-carb days. Good fats and proteins provide you extra energy and facilitate the carb cycling process. Make sure your plan includes a decent range of these.

LOW CARB DAYS: HEALTHY DAYS AND PROTEINS

- Poultry
- Fish, especially that
- rich in heart-healthy Omega-3 fats, such as salmon, tuna, and mackerel

Raw dairy products

like goat cheese, feta, and ricotta

Low-fat dairy products
- Nuts and seeds
- Olive oil, palm oil, and

coconut oil

Leafy greens and all non-starchy
- vegetables
- Avocadoes
- Apples and apricots
- Almond butter

UNHEALTHY FATS AND PROTEINS

Grass-fed lean meat Processed meats like
- bacon, pastrami and

  luncheon meats
- Organic eggs Hot dogs and sausage
- Heavy cream and milk
- Peanut butter

Hopefully, you get the idea. You can now start carb cycling and start adding nutritious foods to your meals!

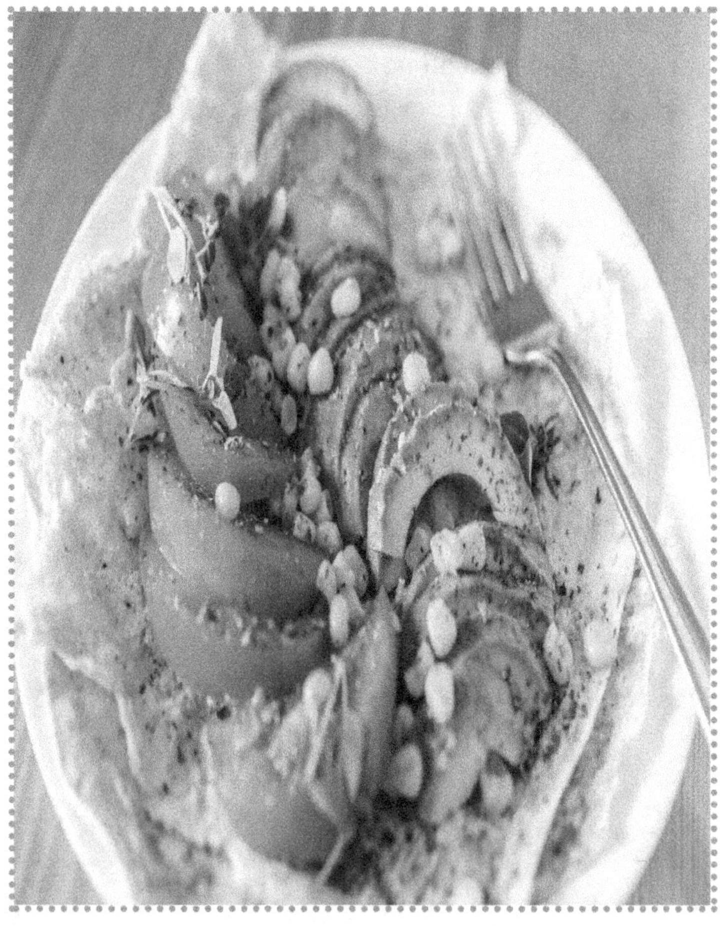

CHAPTER FIVE

Sample Meal Plans

For newbies, it might be intimidating to incorporate all of this knowledge into a detailed meal plan. These meal plans for a typical week of carb cycling are intended to be helpful. Use these as a general guide while creating your meals, but keep in mind that they are not set in stone. Meals can be added or removed based on the seven-day plan that you have selected.

PLAN 1

Monday (low carb day)

Breakfast

• Three entire eggs, fried, cooked, poached, or scrambled.
• 1/2 cup of high-carb fruit like blueberries, pineapple or peaches
• 1/cup oatmeal sweetened with honey

Snack
• I apple or 1/2 cup unsalted nuts

Lunch
• Turkey sandwich with lettuce and tomato on whole- wheat bread.
• Herbal tea

Snack
• 1/2 cup ricotta cheese or 2 medium apricots

Dinner

• Spinach Frittata
• Grilled beef strips with green bell peppers
• Green salad

Tuesday (High carb day)

Breakfast

• Two slices whole wheat bread with Swiss cheese
• 1 cup low-fat yogurt with fresh blueberries

Snack
• 1 banana

Lunch
• Grilled salmon with brown rice
• Grated carrot and cucumber salad

Snack

• 1 slice whole wheat bread with almond butter

Dinner
• Whole wheat pasta with fresh tomatoes
• Black beans with garlic oil
• Fresh green salad

Wednesday (low carb day)

Breakfast

• 3 scrambled eggs with avocado

Snack
• 2 apricots or 2 plums

Lunch
• Caesar salad with grilled chicken strips

• Herbal tea

Snack
• Low-fat yogurt or 1/2 cup of nuts

Dinner
• Steak on the flank with onions and green beans
• Green salad with feta cheese

Thursday (High carb day)

Breakfast

• 2 poached eggs
• 2 slices whole-wheat toast
• 1/2 cup fruit

Snack

• 1/2 cup fruit or nuts or 1 banana

Lunch

• 1 cup brown rice with chickpeas

• Sweet potatoes

• Green salad

Snack

• One banana or low-fat yoghurt with honey

Dinner

• Baked potato

• Grilled chicken breast

• Avocado and tomato salad

Friday (low carb day)

Breakfast

- 1/2 cup oatmeal
- 1/2 cup fruit
- 1/2 cup ricotta, feta or goat cheese

Snack

- 1/2 cup fruit or nuts or 1 low-fat yogurt

Lunch

- Avocado and chicken salad
- Sliced tomatoes on lettuce
- Herbal tea

Snack

- 1 orange or 1 apple or 2 plums

Dinner

• Grilled salmon with vegetables
• beans
• Green salad

Saturday (high carb day)

Breakfast

• 2 scrambled eggs on whole-wheat toast
• 1 low-fat yogurt sweetened with honey

Lunch

• Sweet potatoes
• Lentil soup

Snack

• 1/2 cup nuts or fruit

Dinner

• Tuna Casserole Whole wheat noodles
• Spinach salad

Sunday (low carb + cheat day)

Breakfast

• Lean sausages with fried eggs
• 1/2 cup fruit

Snack

• Almond butter or 1/2 cup nuts

Lunch

• Tuna salad
• 1 piece of fresh fruit

Snack

• 2 plums, two apricots or 1 apple

Dinner

whatever you'd like! Please, in moderation. Have
two slices of pizza, for instance, as opposed to two
or three. Enjoy a small amount of cake or ice cream.
Eat a little plate of French fries rather than a big
platter if you've been desiring them all week. You
understand.

PLAN 2

Here is an example plan to help you if you choose to eat more than three meals a day.

TYPICAL LOW CARB DAY

Meal 1

- 3 egg
- 3 strips of lean bacon
- Sautéed peppers

Meal 2

- 4 oz. grilled turkey or chicken breast
- 1 cup carrots
- Lettuce and tomato salad

Meal 3

- 4 oz grilled salmon, tuna or shrimp
- 1 cup broccoli
- 1 banana

Meal 4

- 4 oz. chicken
- 1 cup spinach
- 1 low-fat yogurt with honey

Meal 5

- 4 oz. tuna
- 1 cup chickpeas
- 1 sliced tomato or cucumber

Meal 6

- 4 oz. lean steak
- 1 cup green beans
- 1/2 cup fruit

TYPICAL HIGH CARB DAY

Meal 1

- 2 eggs
- Three little sausages or three bacon strips
- 2 slices whole-wheat toast

Meal 2

- 4 oz. chicken
- Green salad
- 1/2 cup oatmeal sweetened with honey

Meal 3

- 4 oz. salmon
- 1/2 cup brown rice
- 1/2 cup carrots and peas

Meal 4

- 4 oz. chicken
- 2 cups spinach
- 1 cup arb-rich fruit like peaches, plums or apricots

Meal 5

- 1 cup of corn
- 1 sliced cucumber
- Half a cup of quinoa or wild rice

Meal 6

- 4 oz. grilled beefsteak

- 1 yam
- 1 cup green beans
- Green salad

PLAN 3

Here's a third sample meal plan that merely gives you a few ideas per day so you can use the portion calculations you learned in the last chapter.
Low carb day

Breakfast

- Egg muffins
- Sour cream with chives
- 1 banana

OR...

- Whole wheat pancakes with cream cheese
- 3 sausages
- Blueberries or diced pineapple

OR...

- Three scrambled eggs topped with tomatoes and green peppers
- Vanilla yogurt with sliced banana

Lunch

- Tacos with lean ground beef
- Green salad
- 1 piece whole fruit

OR...

- Lean ground beef stuffing within bell peppers
- Sliced cucumber and spinach topped with grated parmesan cheese
- 1 apple

OR...

• Chicken salad on lettuce

• Baked butternut squash with herbs

• Fruit salad

Dinner

• Grilled chicken pieces and parmesan cheese
paired with whole wheat spaghetti

• Green beans with carrots

• Oatmeal sweetened with honey

OR...

• Beef stroganoff with mushrooms

• Brown rice

• Shredded lettuce and tomato salad

• Jelly cup

OR...

• Chicken fajita wraps

• Zucchini boats stuffed with mozzarella

• Green salad

• 1 piece whole fruit

Snacks

• Rice cake with almond butter

• Protein shake

• Hummus dip and celery sticks

• Strawberry and banana smoothie

• Cottage cheese with honey

• Cream cheese with herbs and carrot sticks

HIGH CARB DAYS

Breakfast

• Scrambled eggs with bacon and chives
• Oatmeal with blueberries and honey
• 1 piece whole fruit

OR...

• Boiled eggs
• 2 slices whole-wheat bread with cream cheese

• 1 banana

OR...

• Fried eggs with sausage
• 2 slices whole wheat toast
• 1 yam

Lunch

• Grilled turkey sandwich
• Chickpea salad
• Yogurt with honey

OR...

• Grilled salmon
• Sweet potato and spinach salad
• 1 piece whole fruit

OR...

- Shrimp with whole wheat noodles
- Potato salad
- 1 piece whole fruit

Dinner:

- Baked chicken
- Mexican brown rice
- Peas with carrots
- 1 piece whole fruit

OR...

- Pan steak with potatoes
- Broccoli with sweet corm
- Jelly cup

OR...

• Pasta with chicken and mushroom

• Cherry tomato and spinach salad

• Quinoa sweetened with honey

As you can see, there's enough space to be inventive and cook delectable food. Once you get the hang of it, you'll be able to whip up delectable sweets that the whole family will appreciate (though youngsters and family members who aren't following the plan shouldn't count calories or portions).

You can also tweak your favorite recipes to make them carb cycling-friendly by replacing processed carbs with healthy ones, and saturated fats with good fats.

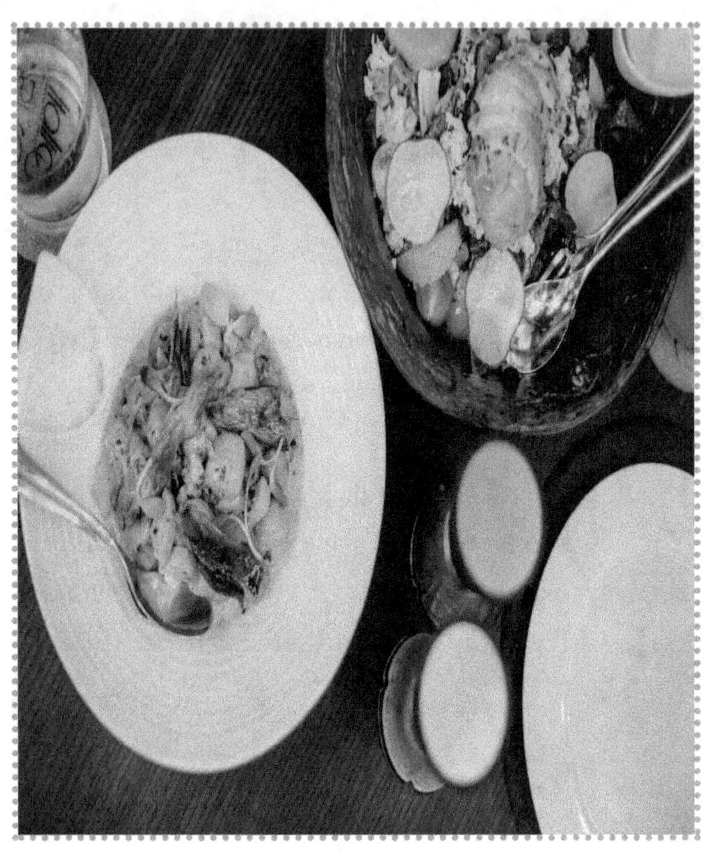

CHAPTER SIX

Typical Side Effects to Anticipate

Remain calm. The adverse effects don't pose any threat at all. Think of them as mild symptoms that could be uncomfortable.

Any abrupt dietary or exercise regimen adjustments could have some short-term negative effects. It is comparable to working out after being inactive for a while. Afterward, your muscles will hurt for a few days. But you're aware that it's because of your exercise.

A few individuals who began the carb cycling regimen have mentioned that they had some negative side effects. These should go away in a week or so, or drastically diminish.

1. Increased water weight. You should anticipate gaining some water weight, particularly on days when you consume a lot of carbohydrates. This is due to the fact that for every gram of carbohydrates

you eat, your body stores four times as much water. With time, this ought to become normal.

On low-carb days, you'll notice less weight gain from water. You can be confident that you are not actually gaining weight.

On days with a lot of carbohydrates, exercising might also be helpful. It should be noted that you still need to drink a lot of water throughout the day in spite of this water weight gain.

2. The first week or so may find you feeling more exhausted and drowsy than normal. This is typical. Once the glucose cycling starts, you'll feel more energized than before, if not more so than normal.

3. Bloating or constipation are possible. Your heavy consumption of carbohydrates—especially from starchy meals like rice and potatoes—is the cause of this.

Herbal teas are a great remedy for this, chamomile tea in particular. Until your digestion is better, you can also substitute stewed fruit for the fruit you normally eat.

4. You might feel agitated and go through mood fluctuations. This is a typical grievance.It's possible that the carb cycling diet is too restrictive for you. What is meant by that? You are restricting yourself if you typically eat more carbohydrates than what this plan calls for. For the first few days following this deprivation, there may be some irritation and moodiness.

5. When you transition from unhealthy to good fats and carbohydrates, you could have cravings. You can overcome this with the assistance of your willpower and cheat day.

6. On low-carb days, your body could need more carbohydrates.

With the exception of the previously mentioned benign side effects, there is actually no risk associated with a carb cycling diet. But always pay attention to what your body is telling you. You might not be a good candidate for the carb diet if these adverse effects persist for longer than two weeks.

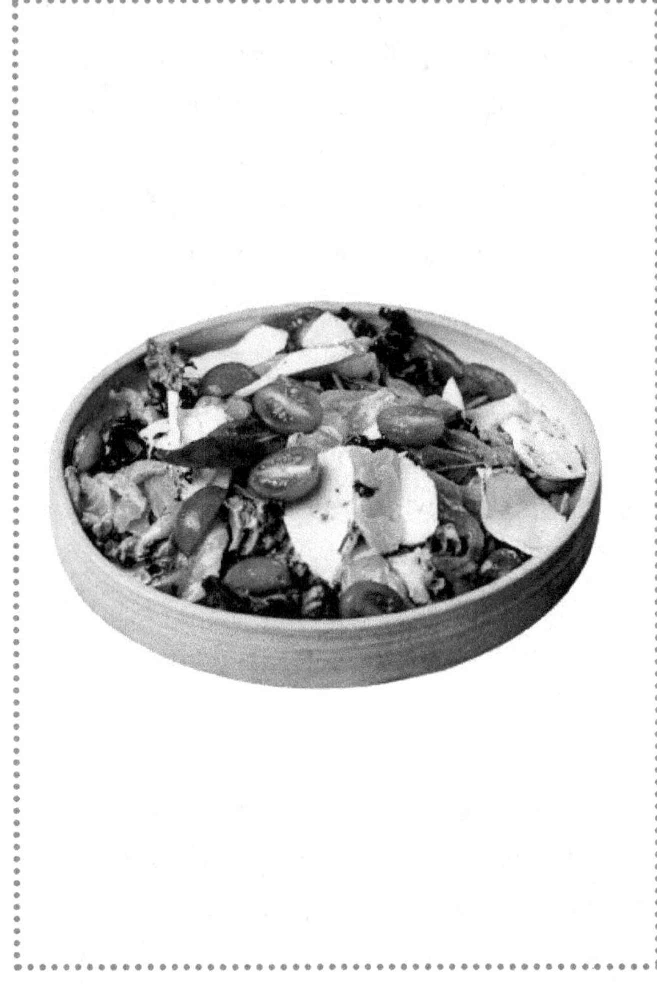

CHAPTER SEVEN

Practical Advice

Here are some practical suggestions to increase the efficacy of your carb cycling program. You could already be working on a few of these.

1. Cheat days don't serve as an excuse to overindulge in all of your favorite foods. If you're truly desiring pizza, have a slice or a Big Mac. Just keep in mind that the cheat day is a choice rather than a must.

How much you "cheat" will determine how well your carb cycling goes. It goes without saying that your weight loss will be slower if you do it every week. Reduce the number of cheat days if you want faster results.

2. Eat a healthy breakfast every day that includes both protein and fiber. This is crucial to squelching

your desires and sustaining your fullness until your next meal.

3. To preserve your muscle mass and maximize carb cycling, think about resistance or aerobic training. You can benefit from any exercise you choose if this doesn't appeal to you. Swimming, cycling, and walking are suitable substitutes.

4. If you exercise frequently or participate in sports, plan your high-carb days to coincide with your high-activity days. This will enable you to lose weight more quickly. On those days, your energy levels will also be higher.

5. Steer clear of "drinking" calories. This covers fruit juices, coffee, tea that has been sweetened, and smoothies. Remain with herbal teas or water. Try to have your coffee black in the morning if you must have it. When tea is sweetened with honey, it doesn't taste all that horrible.

6. Supplements can help with digestion and keep your carb cycling at its ideal level. Probiotics, vitamin B12, and omega-3 are excellent options.

7. Be imaginative when creating menus. Utilize your extensive food assortment to make delectable delicacies. Look for new recipes online and play around with different carb combinations. Additionally, try out items you've never tried anything like hummus, quinoa, or greens. It might surprise you in a good way!

8. Get enough rest to maintain your energy and prevent stress. Let your body recover so that you can engage in healthy carb cycling. This makes perfect sense for everyone who wants to improve their health.

Conclusion

This was a straightforward explanation of the principles behind the carb diet. Everything you require to get started has been provided.

What are the key lessons learned, then?

• The way carb cycling functions is by boosting your metabolism to burn fat and gain muscle at the same time.
• The seven-day schedule that forms the basis of carb cycling alternates high-carb and low-carb days.
• You organize your meals according to the daily allowance of carbohydrates, proteins, and fats.
• You reduce your weight!
Carb-free diets aren't effective for everyone.
There may be too much cravings as a result of the deprivation.

The 7-day carb cycling diet is not restrictive, therefore your chances of following it are significantly increased. You can still eat carbohydrates on low-carb days. This may be the simplest and least uncomfortable method of weight loss.

It's worth a try if you find the flexibility and large selection of dishes intriguing. It is undoubtedly far less inflexible and limiting, and many have said they barely ever get hungry. Of course, the biggest advantage is gaining muscle mass and decreasing weight at the same time. So go ahead, load up on lean proteins and carbohydrates, enjoy creating your meal plans, and begin feeling, looking, and becoming in better shape right now.

www.ingramcontent.com/pod-product-compliance
Lightning Source LLC
Chambersburg PA
CBHW051655250726
48653CB00007B/2672